MW01132255

First published in the UK in 2018 by Peter Regan

Copyright © 2018 Peter Regan

About the Author

In 1973 Peter Regan began his hairdressing career in Central Manchester. In 1976 he joined Vidal Sassoon and worked his way up to become a member of the UK Artistic Team. In 1982 he moved on from Vidal Sassoon and forged a successful career in the British Film Industry. Following a period studying prosthetics, first at Berlin University and later with Christopher Tucker (creator of the Elephant Man), he worked for a number of years as a Chief Hair and Make-up Artist in charge of the hair and make-up departments on numerous feature film and television productions. In 2000 he opened his own salon in Central Manchester, where he still sees clients on a daily basis.

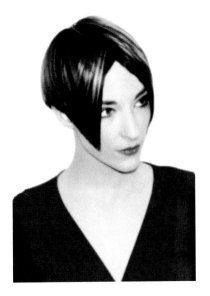

The Hair Colour Book

Welcome to The Hair Colour Book, a practical guide to the theory of colouring hair. We have kept the pure science content to a minimum, as it can be distracting. Instead we have concentrated on the practical aspects of colouring hair, in plain and simple English. This book is a resource that can be used for reference as well as a clear explanation of the theory.

This book contains a number of sections which contain information relating to their particular subject. Each has a check-list at the end so that you can find the information easily. The third part is a quick reference guide, where you can see in a sentence, information which can be used to jog your memory. The final part is the Glossary where terms used in the book are listed in alphabetical order along with an explanation.

CONTENTS

THE CONSULTATION

The first task. Find out about the customer's hair and what they want.

Whenever a customer books for a colour service for the first time, colourists should always conduct a skin compatibility evaluation (Patch Test). It is required for all new customers and those who have not had their hair coloured in your salon in the last 6 months and should be performed no less than 48 hours prior to the application of colour.

Check the following with the customer:

Have they ever had an allergic reaction to any hair colourant product?

An allergic reaction to any kind of skin tattoo including Henna or to permanent make-up

Do they have a sensitive, irritated or damaged scalp? (e.g. eczema or psoriasis)

Have they been prescribed and are taking any medication to treat allergies?

If your customer answers YES to any of these questions then you should not colour their hair until they first check with their doctor. Even regular customers should be asked if they have had any of the above since their last visit, if they have, then another skin test should be performed.

All hair is different. At the consultation we may be looking at a head of hair that has been previously coloured at home and now has a mixture of virgin hair at the root, then a gradual build-up, of colour towards the ends. Another customer may have had some old bleach highlights coloured over and has decided she wants to go lighter again. Each customer's hair has its own set of features which need to be looked at on an individual basis. Sometimes the practicalities mean that we have to advise the customer that their original idea is not possible because the risk of damage is too great. Damaging the customer's hair is simply not acceptable and must be avoided.

Check to see if the customer has had any other processes on the hair previously, perms, straighteners, highlights, all over colours or bleach.

Is the hair porous? If it is, it will need to be treated in a specific way to ensure that the colour is not washed straight out. We'll look at this more detail later.

Does she use heated tools on a regular basis? Blow-driers and straightening/curling irons used too frequently can make the hair very dry and porous and can even cause breakage. This will have a negative effect on the colour's staying power.

How often does she shampoo? Daily shampooing will clearly have more of an effect on the colour than shampooing twice a week.

Look for poor colour work. Examine the hair for any pre-existing colour work. If there are any problems e.g. over-processed bleach, poor coverage or damage, make sure you tell and show this to the customer. This will guarantee that the blame for these problems does not fall to you.

Determine the percentage of white (unpigmented) hair. 25%, 50%, 75% or 100%. White hair can be very resistant, making it difficult to colour. Normal white hair has a coarse slightly rough texture, whilst resistant white hair is smooth and glossy. If there is resistant white hair then additional base will be required in the formulation to ensure coverage.

Determine the texture. Is the hair coarse, average or fine? Hair colour is manufactured to work best on average texture and porosity.

Establish the hair's racial type, natural colour level and tone. Don't rely on guess work, get the colour chart and place it as close as possible to any virgin hair. Don't forget that the top and front are likely to be lighter than the back because they are exposed to external factors (sunlight etc.) that can cause them to fade. Level is the depth of colour (dark v light) and tone is the amount of warmth or coolness that a colour displays. Also check the skin tone and eye colour, is it warm or cool? As experience is gained, the consultation becomes almost automatic. However, it is still important to make sure that you have all of the information required to make the correct colour choices.

Discuss the customer's requirements. It's important to guide them towards colours that will work for their hair's condition, texture and level, if we try to lift the hair too far we could cause damage. Make notes about what you have agreed with the customer and any ideas about the colours you are going to use and what result you expect to get. Make sure that you have recorded the skin test date and product used.

Explain the level of maintenance the colour will require, recommend products for home use and the cost for the service and any ongoing costs for the future.

Once you have agreed with your customer what you are going to do, then simply carry out the plan. It's a good idea to make notes at the time, they should be to the point and accurate. Also make a note of the result, your opinion and the customer's reaction. This will be useful for future visits.

Consultation Check-list:

If it was required, make sure that a skin evaluation test has been carried out according to your manufacturer's instructions.

Check if the customer has virgin hair, previously coloured hair/perm/straightener or any other chemical process.

Identify the hair's racial type.

Check the texture and porosity of the hair. Does she use heated tools that can affect the porosity?

Check the customer's natural level.

Check for white hair, what is the percentage and is it resistant or not.

Decide if semi-permanent, quasi/demi-permanent or permanent colour is required.

If permanent, agree the desired/target level with the customer and note what the exposed contributing pigment will be.

Do you need to neutralise warmth or enhance the exposed contributing pigment?

Advise the customer of the tonal requirements to achieve the desired colour.

LEVELS AND TONES

The simple equation for a hair colour result is:

Contributing pigment + Artificial colour = Final result

To understand this statement, first examine the basic hair colour terms.

Base Colour

The dominant colour in any formulation that gives a shade its overall characteristic regardless of tone.

Level

The degree of lightness or darkness (natural or artificial).

Tone

The warmth or coolness of a colour – warm tones reflect light and make the hair appear lighter, cool tones absorb light and appear darker.

To formulate a hair colour successfully, we must determine the starting, natural base colour and tone, the desired level and tone (finished result). The colour wheel can be used to establish which colours will enhance or neutralise the tones to help us reach our desired or target result.

To fully grasp the workings of the colour wheel, examine the interaction of **Natural Levels, Contributing Pigments** and **Exposed Contributing Pigments.**

Natural Levels

In the UK we identify 10 natural levels of hair colour. Some brands start at level 1 others at level 2. For the purpose of this chapter we will use the level 1 start point. Level 1 is Black. Levels 2-5 are Brown (level 2 is darkest brown), 6-10 are Blonde (level 10 is lightest blonde). There are tints that can be used to change a natural colour to each of these levels depending on the developer used. There is also an extra level, Special (high lift) Blonde. High lift colours are designed to enable hair more than 3 levels darker to be lifted up to level 10. To avoid damaging the hair, we should not lift the hair more than 3-4 levels.

Contributing Pigment

Each natural level has its own contributing pigments sometimes called underlying/residual warmth. This underlying warmth is exposed during the lightening process, giving predictable levels of residual red, orange and yellow which will be left in the hair depending the amount of lift achieved.

Exposed Contributing Pigment

Is the colour that is left after the hair has been lifted to a particular level. If we start with a base level 5 (light brown) and aim to achieve level 7 (medium blonde) the residual colour left behind will be *yellow orange*. Level 8 will leave *yellow*, and so on. The colour can be enhanced or neutralised by choosing the correct tone depending on our desired result. Below is a table showing what the Exposed Contributing Pigments are at each level.

NATURAL LEVEL	EXPOSED CONTRIBUTING PIGMENT
10 - Lightest Blonde	VERY PALE YELLOW
9 - Very Light Blonde	PALE YELLOW
8 - Light Blonde	YELLOW
7 - Medium Blonde	YELLOW ORANGE
6 - Dark Blonde	ORANGE
5 - Light Brown	REDDISH ORANGE
4 - Medium Brown	REDDISH BROWN
3 - Dark Brown	BROWN
2 - Darkest Brown	DARK BROWN
1 - Black	BLACK

The Shade Chart

The swatches in your shade chart indicate the colours that are available within the range. They are grouped in families. For example, there will be Natural/Neutral shades, Golds, Browns, Reds and High Lift, each manufacturer refers to them slightly differently. The Natural/Neutral family are your base colours. They can be added to other colours to intensify and assist in coverage of white hair, or other colours can be added to them to increase, neutralise or enhance tone. Double bases are used exclusively for coverage of resistant white hair.

When using the shade chart don't forget that you can only achieve lift at the levels that your chosen hydrogen peroxide will allow (see "Developers and Mixing" page 69).

Levels and Tones Check-list:

Make sure you understand the equation for a hair colour result.

Contributing pigment + Artificial colour = Final result

Understand the relationship between natural level and desired/target level.

Know what colours are exposed after you lift the hair.

Use the colour wheel to assist in choosing the correct tones to either neutralise or enhance.

Understand your shade chart and use it to find the precise colours you need to create your formula.

The Colour Wheel

Formulating hair colour can be a bit daunting. Before starting any colour, take a moment to consider the colour wheel. When you understand how it works, you can combine this knowledge with the other elements of formulation (base level, desired level and tone) and make the right choice of colour for the formula.

The Colour Wheel

The rules of the colour wheel are simple and they are the same if you're an artist working in oil paint on canvas, or a hair colourist creating great hair colour. Here are the three most important things we need to know about the colour wheel.

One:

There are three primary colours, RED, YELLOW and BLUE; they are the foundation of all the colours we see.

Two:

There are three secondary colours, produced when you mix equal parts of two primary colours, GREEN (yellow and blue), VIOLET (blue and red) and ORANGE (red and yellow).

Three:

There are six tertiary colours. These are created by mixing equal parts of one primary colour and one secondary colour. YELLOW-GREEN (**yellow** and green), BLUE-GREEN (**blue** and green), BLUE-VIOLET (**blue** and violet), RED-VIOLET (**red** and violet), RED-ORANGE (**red** and orange) and YELLOW-ORANGE (**yellow** and orange). The primary colour is always placed first as it is the dominant colour.

The Colour Wheel

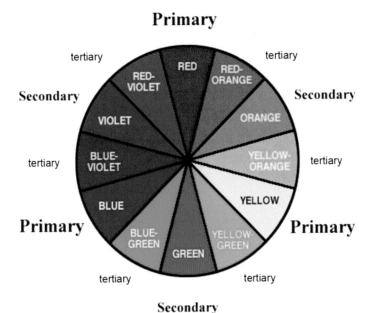

Next, residual colour after lifting. For colour ranges that start at level 1, number the segments on the wheel as follows: (1) Blue, (2) Blue/Violet, (3) Violet, (4) Red/Violet, (5) Red, (6) Red/Orange, (7) Orange (8) Yellow/Orange, (9) Yellow and (10) Pale Yellow. For ranges that start at level 2, move forward one segment as level 1 is absent e.g. level 2 becomes violet and so on. Each number represents a level. This means that if we start with a natural level 5 and want to lift the colour to natural looking level 7, the exposed contributing pigment (residual colour) will be Orange (or Yellow/Orange for ranges starting at level 2).

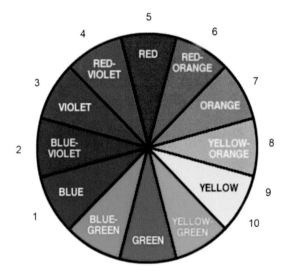

Colour wheel showing residual colours after lifting to a specific level

To neutralise the residual tone, we must use the opposite colour on the wheel, in this case blue (or blue-violet). Whatever the blue tones are in the colour you use, the effect achieved will be to bring the colour back to a level 7 brown. The amount of lift possible is determined by the natural level and the strength of hydrogen peroxide used. We will discuss developers a little later in this book.

The Colour Wheel Check-list:

Make sure to consult your colour wheel.

Remember all colours are made from the three primary colours.

Primary, secondary and tertiary colours are used for controlling tone.

Use the residual colour wheel to identify the residual colour at a specific level.

THE NUMBERING SYSTEM

Each colour manufacturer uses their own unique numbering system. These are the numbers in the colour charts or on the end of the boxes and refer to the depth and tone of the product. There are numbers with a slash, comma, hyphen or dot in-between them, this is called a separator. Sometimes there is no separator but a letter after the depth number. Letters like N for natural or G for gold are used. Some manufacturers start at level 1 others at level 2.

Wella Koleston Perfect	L'Oreal Majirel	Schwartzkopf Igora Royal	Clynol Viton S	Goldwell Topchic
33/0	3	3-0	3-0	3N
7/07	7.0	7-7	7.03	7B
6/1	6.1	6-2	6.1	6A

Most brands do use a separator, the numbers to the left represent the depth of the colour (level). Double numbers tell us there is an extra portion of the base colour in this product.

These are the levels when the chart starts at Level 1:

1 Black

2 Very Dark Brown

3 Dark Brown

4 Medium Brown

5 Light Brown

6 Dark Blonde

7 Medium Blonde

8 Light Blonde

9 Very Light Blonde

10 Lightest Blonde

These are the levels when the chart starts at Level 2:

2 Black

3 Dark Brown

4 Medium Brown

5 Light Brown

6 Dark Blonde

7 Medium Blonde

8 Light Blonde

9 Very Light Blonde

10 Lightest Blonde

The numbers to the right of the separator describe the tone. Because there is so much variation, it's important that you find out as much as you can about the colour range that you are using. Also, some manufacturers supply more than one range and these can also have different numbering systems. Look underneath the swatch in your colour chart, there should be a description of the colour. Normal bases will say something like "Light Blonde" or "Medium Brown", those that add "Deep" or "Intense" are used to for extra coverage on resistant white hair. Most brands use a similar description for the depth of their colours. Just check your colour chart, they are usually referred to as "Basic" or "Naturals".

The tonal numbers are less straight forward, we know that these describe the tone but here the manufacturers differ in their descriptions. Wella calls /7 "Brown" whilst L'oreal calls their .7 "Green Metallic". You just need to learn your brand and follow a few simple rules. The brands that use letters instead of numbers should be treated the same way.

The first number to the right of the separator is the dominant tone, if there is just one character then that will be the only tone included. If there are 2 characters then the second is the minor tone and will be less visible than the dominant tone. Generally, there will be twice as much dominant tone to minor tone. However, it will still have an effect on the result. Here is the International Colour Chart tonal system. You can see that the number relates to a tone, the actual colour the tone belongs to and whether it is cool or warm.

ICC Number Tone Actual Colour Cool or Warm

.1 Blue Ash Blue Cool

.2 Mauve Ash Purple Cool

.3 Gold Yellow Warm

.4 Copper Orange Warm

.5 Mahogany Red/Violet Neutral

.6 Red Red Warm

.7 Khaki Green Cool

20

.8 Pearl Ash Cool

.9 Soft Ash Cool

.0- – – Cool

.-0 – – Depends on dominant tone

The Numbering System Check-list:

The separator identifies the level to the left and the tone to the right.

Double numbers to the left (88/--) tell us it is for covering resistant white hair.

The tones to the right are used to neutralise or enhance residual warmth at our desired level.

See which numbers and tones go together in your colour chart.

RACIAL DIFFERENCES IN HAIR

It's quite simple to tell the differences in the three main hair types, look below at the cross section and distribution of the pigment granules.

African hair is thin and almost flat in cross section. It is defined by very tight curls and is the slowest growing of the hair types at about 0.9cm per month. The angle of growth is nearly parallel to the scalp. Nearly always very dark brown or black, the pigment granules are densely packed throughout the cortex and around the medulla.

African hair: It has a coarse cuticle and a flat shape. Extremely curly, it is densely pigmented throughout the cortex, making it more difficult to colour.

Asian hair: Hair shaft has a larger diameter, straight and is almost perfectly round. Pigment granules are large and are distributed throughout the cortex. Difficult to lift due to density of colour

European hair: Slightly oval in shape, has the widest variation of pigment and texture. Straight to wavy, fine to thick. The colour granules are distributed close to the cuticle, making it easier to lift and colour.

The combination of texture and density of colour granules makes African hair very resistant to artificial colour.

Asian hair is circular in cross section, although not perfectly. It is the fastest growing hair type at 1.3cm per month. It grows out of the scalp at a right angle and the colour granules are densely distributed throughout the cortex. It is nearly always naturally black in colour and tends to be straight.

European hair grows out of the scalp at an oblique angle - not parallel and not at a right angle. It is oval in cross section and has the most varied range of natural textures and colours. Growing at about 1.2cm per month the pigment granules are sparse to moderately distributed mainly around the inside of the cuticle. It is the easiest hair type to colour.

African type hair is very curly making it difficult apply the colour evenly, it is also difficult to see exactly where the colour is being applied. Try straightening the hair before colouring, this will enable you to coat the hair uniformly and place the colour exactly where you want it to be. You will also use less formula, reducing waste.

The darker the hair the more difficult it will be to lift without damage. African, Asian and some European hair types are extremely dark and hard to lift. These hair types are rarely able to lift beyond 3-4 levels and will always expose a lot of warmth.

As you can see in the illustration on page 34, both African and Asian hair have a large amount of pigment which is found deep inside the hair shaft. This is what makes this type of hair harder to colour as it is more difficult to lift out enough of the existing colour granules to allow the new colour to be deposited. Lifting the hair more than 3-4 levels may cause damage and the result may not be satisfactory. The difference to both the original colour and skin tone will be too great and the exposed contributing pigment will be unattractive.

European hair is the easiest to colour as there is less dark pigment and it is found closer to the cuticle, making it easier to oxidise the colour granules and deposit the new colour into the cortex.

Racial Differences in Hair Check-list:

Remember, the darker the hair the more difficult it will be to lift.

African type hair has a coarse irregular texture and requires a larger amount of product.

Very dark hair has a large amount of dark pigment, meaning it cannot be successfully lifted beyond 3-4 levels and will expose warmth.

European hair is the easiest to colour, as there is less dark pigment to deal with.

CONTROLLING WARMTH

Whenever we lighten hair, we leave behind a residual colour. We discussed it earlier - "Exposed Contributing Pigment". If the hair is dark, there is always an underlying red pigment that is concealed, giving depth to brown hair. When we lighten it with tint or bleach, we reveal this residual tone, known as warmth. As we saw from the colour wheel, all colours are a mixture of red, yellow and blue. Blue has the largest colour molecule and is the easiest to remove and when the blue is gone that leaves red and yellow. When red and yellow are mixed together we see orange. Red is next, leaving just yellow behind. Hair undergoes different levels of red through to orange and finally yellow, the more we lighten it. This is why we have to create a formula for each individual customer that takes into consideration each element required to create a successful colour. As mentioned previously the equation is *"Contributing pigment + Artificial colour = Final result"*.

Here's an example. A customer who is a natural level 7 and wants to be a level 10 natural looking blonde. The hair needs to be lifted by 3 levels to achieve the level required. Use the "Residual Colour Wheel" that shows exposed colour after lifting, it shows that the natural undertone at level 7 (Medium Blonde) is orange/yellow (gold). However, you will see that when it reaches level 10 the hair will be showing an exposed very pale yellow colour. This means that the blue and the majority of red pigment have been lifted out. This yellow does not give us the natural blonde look we are aiming for, so we must add something into the formula to correct the tone. As we are lifting from level 7 to level 10 bleach is not required, so a level 10 tint with a violet tone (remember the characters to the right of the separator --/--) will be required. This will neutralise the yellow and give the shade of blonde that is the target colour.

Warmth is the amount of red, red/yellow pigment left in the hair following a lifting process. It is controlled by correctly using the colour wheel to identify the exact tones present and the tones required to either neutralise or enhance. Opposites neutralise and neighbours enhance.

So far, we have been dealing with virgin hair. What if the hair has been previously coloured? It could be lighter than the natural level or it could be darker. What if there is a re-growth? The way you handle previously processed hair is vitally important to the finished result. Unless the customer has experienced a colour disaster, which would probably mean some form of colour correction is required; it is likely that there will be a re-growth. If we are just doing a root touch-up, all we need to do is follow the normal rules of colouring, *Contributing pigment + Artificial colour = Final result*.

The same rules apply for darkening the hair, except it is important to assess the porosity of the previously lightened hair. If the hair shows signs of damage and looks faded it is probably porous. Depending on the extent, a mix tone should be added to the formula or a filler (recipe on page 61) will be required. This is to replace the missing tones from the hair and make the colour hold. If there is a re-growth, depending on porosity and condition, we may need to use two different colours along with the added tone for the porous hair to achieve a satisfactory result.

Controlling Warmth Check-list

Always check the natural level.

Always check what the Exposed Contributing Pigment will be at your target level.

Know what pigment will remain after each level is achieved.

Know what effect previously tinted hair will have.

Use the colour wheels to identify neutralising and enhancing tones.

ADDING TONE

Most of the colours in your colour chart are pre-mixed base and tone. You can use them to achieve most of the colours you will ever need. However, they are not the only way to add tone to your colours. Usually found at the back of the colour chart you will find the special mix colours. Also known as mix-tones, these products are pure tone and can be used to intensify a colour or correct a tone. They can also be added in to your tint formula, if the hair is porous, e.g. if you are taking an artificial blonde back to brown and are concerned that the colour won't hold because of porosity. Maybe you are dealing with very dark hair that has a lot of red undertone and you may feel that the pre-mixed colours are not strong enough to counteract the orange that will be exposed as you lift the hair. With these colours you can select something to add to your formula that will replace or correct the tone, giving you the colour, you were aiming for.

Usually grouped warm and cool, they will enable you to make all of the tones within the colour chart (remember tones are to the right of the separator). Because mix-tones can be used to create the pre-mixed colours when combined with a base colour, you can use them to make colours if you do not have the pre-mixed colour available. They can be used on pre-bleached hair to create exceptional, vibrant colours and can be added to toners to help correct unwanted tone.

Refer to your colour chart for the correct mixing ratio for your product. Some brands refer to mix-tones with numbers that relate to the normal tones in the chart. Others call them Red, Green or Blue etc.

Adding Tone Checklist:

Find the special mix/mix-tone colours at the back of your shade chart.

Don't forget they are pure tone and need to be handled according to the manufacturer's instructions.

You can make colours if the pre-mixed colour is not available.

They can be used to create vibrant, bright colours.

GREY COVERAGE

Before creating a formula to cover grey hair, we should first take a moment to look at a few facts about grey hair and what grey hair is. Firstly, there is no such thing as an actual grey hair. Non-pigmented hairs are white. As we age, some hair follicles stop producing the pigment melanin. Melanin is required to give the hair its colour. Either the individual hairs lose their ability to create pigment and grow white from the hair follicle, or they are simply new hairs that do not contain pigment. As it is rare for all of the hairs to become white, there will be a mixture of darker and white hairs mixed together. When this happens, the white hair dilutes the dark appearance of the hair and the overall look is grey. With natural redheads, the colour can dilute to a strawberry blonde. White hair is much less obvious in naturally blonde hair. The more of the non-pigmented hair there is, the whiter the hair will look.

In most salons the most popular colour service is covering white hair in one way or another. All over colours being the most obvious but highlights are often used to blend in white hairs and semi-permanent colours are used for people with a lesser amount of white hair. Another popular service is a mixture of an all over tint combined with highlights. As we can see, there are quite a few services that we can offer to our customers to blend or cover unwanted white hair. Let's take a look at what they do and how they work.

Most hair colourant manufacturers refer to their products by levels.

Level 1:

Semi-permanent colour - true semi-permanent colours are not activated by Hydrogen Peroxide and are not oxidative. They coat the cuticle of the hair and are used to make the hair darker or stay at the same depth, they cannot lighten the hair and do not hold fast. Typically, they last for 4 to 6 washes and will not damage the hair.

Level 2:

Quasi semi-permanent sometimes called demi colours or mildly oxidising colours, cannot be washed out, rather they fade out gradually due to exposure to daylight (UV) and washing. Unlike Level 3 colourants, they do not contain ammonia which makes them less permanent. They sit just underneath the cuticle and do not fully penetrate the cortex. Coverage is in the region of up to 40% white/grey hair and they last for up to 20 washes. Care should be taken to ensure the correct level of hydrogen peroxide is used, as too high a percentage can make them act like permanent colour and leave a re-growth line.

Level 3:

Permanent colourants. These are the most versatile of all hair colourants, they can lighten, stay at the same level or darken the hair and 100% white coverage can be achieved. The level of lightening is in direct proportion to the strength of the hydrogen peroxide used in the formula. It should be noted that the lighter the hair is lifted, the more damage there is likely to be. These are oxidative colourants, which means that they have the ability to remove natural colour and deposit artificial colour at the same time. This is achieved by the ammonia in the tint cream opening the cuticle and the hydrogen peroxide oxidising the existing colour in the hair, then the pigment granules contained in the cream are deposited into the cortex

Most people, who want to cover white hair, do so in order to keep their natural colour intact. These people are not looking for change. However, some people want to make their hair lighter than their natural colour. It should be noted that you can only achieve 100% coverage of white hair on levels 8 and below.

There are 2 types of white hair - resistant and non-resistant. Non-resistant white hair is slightly coarse in texture and a little wiry looking; it accepts the colour quite readily. Resistant white hair on the other hand is smooth and glossy in appearance as the cuticle is tightly flattened, this makes it difficult for the pigment to penetrate the hair shaft. Some hairdressers advocate pre-softening resistant white hair but this is not an advisable strategy. Pre-softening involves applying neat Hydrogen Peroxide (developer) to the hair and leaving it on the hair for 5-10 minutes to raise the cuticle and make it easier for the colour to take. The hair is then rinsed and dried and finally the colour formula is applied as normal. The problem is this, applying neat developer to the customer's scalp area is potentially harmful and should always be avoided. Instead, add an extra portion of natural base colour to your recipe with 6% developer and ensure that the hair is fully saturated with the formula. Process under heat for the maximum recommended time and then remove from heat and leave for a further 10 minutes. Then remove the colour as normal.

The pigments which give hair its colour are called melanins, there are two different melanins present in all hair types - Eumelanin which is responsible for the brown-black pigment and Phaeomalanin which is responsible for the red-yellow.

How they blend together determines what the colour of the hair will be. White hair is the result of the melanin content of the hair not being present. When the brown-black of the eumelanin and the red-yellow of the phaeomelanin are missing, the hair will become white. Sometimes this happens as the hair is growing but often it happens to new hairs.

When covering white hair, it is best to use the natural/neutral family of tints from your colour palette. Natural/neutral colours are a mixture of red, yellow and blue. Brown is simply equal amounts of these primary colours. Also, natural/neutral colours do not contain additional tone that could give an unwanted result. Certain ash tone products when applied to white hair can give off a violet cast (that is you will see a violet tinge on the hair). If you want to add a little tone to your natural base try adding something like a natural gold to the formula. There are a number of natural tones that you can add just make sure that you understand what colour they will produce. Make sure that the ratio of colours is correct and that your natural base is the main part or the tonal part of the formula will be too dominant.

First determine the amount of white hair present. Don't worry about being precise, up to 25%, 25-50%, 50-75% and 75-100% is fine. Decide which materials are most appropriate level 1 colour (semi-permanent) will not cover much at all, Level 2 colour (quasi or demi colour) will cover about 40% and level 3 (permanent) will cover up to 100%. If the customer has been coming to the salon for a long time, it is likely that as white hairs have appeared they would have tried semi then demi then moved on to permanent colours. New clients are likely to have had some form of colour before coming to your salon. You should make sure that you find out as much as you can about the procedures that have been performed prior to them coming to see you.

1. What previous procedures have been carried out, if any?

2. Has the hair been lightened and then made darker?

3. How well have any previous services worked?

4. Do they want to be lighter than their natural colour or darker?

5. If there is already artificial colour, is it darker or lighter than the natural colour?

6. What level is it and is it even?

7. Is there a re-growth?

8. What is the natural level of the re-growth?

9. Do you need to use more than one formula to achieve your target result because of the difference between the artificial colour and the re-growth?

Examine and determine the current state of the customer's hair.

What is the Natural level? Is there any artificial colour if so what is it and its level? Most customers want to match their own natural colour as closely as possible, so be careful to ensure that you know what their natural level is - use your colour chart, don't guess. Ask colleagues about the characteristics of the brand of colour you are using, some turn out darker or lighter than the colour chart predicts. This will help when you are formulating. Don't forget that the general rule is, "Tint Won't Lift Tint" and therefore if there is any existing artificial colour, you will need to formulate either at the same level or darker. If the desired result is to be lighter, then a colour correction is required and will need to be performed by a colourist with suitable experience.

Decide the Desired Level.

If you are not trying to match your customer's natural colour, you should determine your client's desired level. During your consultation, find out about their desired hair colour, make sure to discuss the level of commitment required to maintain their new look. They should understand from the outset the amount of commitment and maintenance the colour requires.

Determine the required tone.

Once you have determined the level wanted, move on to tone. You should consider your client's skin tone and eye colour. Lighter blue eyes indicate a cooler skin tone, whilst green and brown eyes indicate a warmer tone. Warm complexions have yellow undertones, cool complexions have pink undertones. Although your skin may become lighter or darker depending on how tanned you are, whether deliberate tanning or just from normal exposure to the sun, skin tone will remain constant.

If your customer has virgin hair then it is possible that they wish to be lighter. This can easily be achieved with tint. However, it should be noted that you will only achieve 100% coverage of white hair with tint, at level 8 and below. If there is resistant white hair at the front, apply the tint to this hair first so that it is exposed to the formula for a little longer. Make sure that you apply enough product to fully and evenly saturate the hair; this will ensure an even application and improve the result. The recommended development time can be extended by 10 minutes to allow for a better penetration 35 - 45 minutes. If the hair is particularly resistant, processing with heat is advised to open the cuticle and allow the product to settle into the cortex. Develop for 25 minutes and then allow to cool for 15 minutes before removing.

Grey Coverage Check-list:

Grey hair is actually white.

Level 1 colour is a true Semi-permanent. Does not lighten the hair

Level 2 colour is a Quasi or Demi-permanent. It is mildly oxidising and cannot lighten the hair.

Level 3 colour is Permanent and can be used to lighten the hair.

The level of lightening is in direct proportion to the strength of hydrogen peroxide used.

Check if there is any existing tint. If so, what is the level?

Check if the hair is non-resistant (slightly coarse and wiry) or resistant (smooth and shiny).

For resistant white hair add an extra portion of natural base to your formula. Process for maximum time under heat and leave for an additional 10 minutes without heat.

For particularly resistant white hair, process under heat for 25 minutes and then leave for 15 minutes without heat. This will enable the colour to settle into the hair and hold more easily.

BLONDES - BLEACH OR TINT

The best candidates for all over blonde are level 7 and above. Attempting to achieve an all over blonde on anything darker will result in a brassy yellow, as there will be too much warmth left in the hair after lifting. With that said, there are a couple of other options to help people become blonder. Highlights are always a good option or an all over colour with highlights woven in to lighten the overall look. With highlights, you can always put in a darker tinted light to add definition and break up the look of the blonde, making it less solid and giving an element of movement to the colour.

The two methods of making hair blonder are bleaching and tinting. With bleach, a cream made from bleach and hydrogen peroxide is applied to the hair and processed to the desired level. It is possible to achieve up to 7 levels of lift with bleach. However, any customer asking for this level of lift should be advised of the potential for damage. They should also be informed that the contrast between the re-growth and the bleached hair will be very obvious. When using bleach, it is always advisable to use the lowest strength peroxide possible. The higher the percentage of peroxide used, the faster the bleach will process and the more damage the hair will suffer. Avoid using bleach with hydrogen peroxide above 6%. It's better to us lower strength peroxide and wait for the bleach to process than to try to achieve a fast result that ends up with damage to the customer's hair.

When used as an all over colour on the scalp, cream bleach should be used. Powder and granular bleach are more intense and can have a damaging effect on both the scalp and hair. After bleaching, the hair will probably require a toner in order to even out the tone and give a satisfactory result. Bleach is best used on hair at level 5 and darker, as from level 6; tint will give a better result with much less damage.

The second method is oxidative tint. This is where a chosen colour and tone as described earlier (using the colour wheel) is applied and the hair is lifted to the desired level and either neutralising or enhancing tone is applied at the same time. Here the level of hydrogen peroxide will directly determine the level of lift that can be achieved. As a general rule, 6% will allow the hair to stay at the same depth or go darker; it will also lift 1 level. 9% will lift 2 levels and 12% will lift 3 levels. High lift blonde colours can lift up to 5 levels.

It is not advisable to attempt to take a customer from level 2 or 3 up to level 9 or 10 as the amount of residual warmth left in the hair will be too dominant and difficult to neutralise.

Blondes - Bleach or Tint Check-list

Avoid all over light blonde on anyone naturally darker than level 7.

Advise highlights or a tint with highlights for those clients with darker hair, who want to be lighter.

When using bleach, chose the lowest percentage hydrogen peroxide you can.

At natural level 6, tint will give a better result, unless you are looking for a deliberately bleached look.

BRUNETTES

After black, brown hair is the second most common human hair colour. It varies from light brown to almost black and is right at the centre of our Colour Wheel. Whenever we use neutralising tones in our formulations to control warmth, we are creating brown. It doesn't matter if it is a light creamy blonde or a dark chestnut; it is still primarily a shade of brown.

Why does the customer want to be brunette (or brown)? Has she been blonde for a long time and decided to go back to her natural colour? Does she have naturally very dark hair and wants it to be lighter? Does she have a lot of white hair that has been tinted dark and is finding that it has built up too much?

Let's look at the customer who has been blonde and now wants to go back to her natural colour. As we know from previous sections of this book, in order to become blonde, it is necessary for the natural dark pigment to be removed from the hair. The action of lifting the hair goes through various stages before the desired (target) level is achieved. Some stylists call this, "The Stages of Lift". Starting at level 2 (natural or previously coloured hair) the hair lifts and leaves behind red, then red/orange, then orange, then yellow/orange (gold), then yellow and finally pale yellow. By the time we get to our desired level, all of the previous colours have been removed from the hair. In order to take the hair back from yellow to brown we must first replace the missing tones. In this case, to achieve pale yellow (level 10); all of the reds and oranges are removed, followed by yellow until pale yellow is reached. As we know, yellow and orange make gold and red and yellow make orange. As there is still pale yellow in the hair, we need to replace the red and orange, use the red and orange from the special mix colours from your product company. All colour manufacturers provide special mix colours; they are also called mix-tones. When used they will add back the missing tones, allowing you to create the best canvas to place your target colour on to. Use them in the following way:

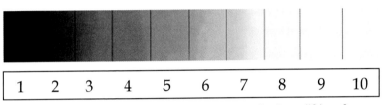

The order that the colours are removed when lifting from very dark to lightest blonde

The diagram on the previous page shows the colours that are removed as we lift the hair. We are starting with a level 10 and a target of level 6. If you just apply the target tint (level 6) to the hair, you will not achieve an evenly distributed colour, it may look patchy if it grabs in some areas but not in others, it will not reach your target colour and will fade very quickly.

We know that the residual or exposed contributing pigment at level 6 is orange (or red/orange, depending on your brand). Sometimes people refer to it as underlying colour. For your information, residual colour and underlying colour are the same thing. In this case, the tones which need to be replaced are red and orange. The special mix colours used are all the same in all of the ranges of colour that are professionally available. However, each manufacturer refers to them differently. Some use numbers to describe the mix tones i.e. Wella calls the mix tone we need 0/43 this is because on the tonal side of the separator the 4 stands for red and the 3 stands for orange, L'oreal will call the colour copper as copper is a mixture of red and orange The identity of the colour required will depend on the brand you use. Just find out from your colour chart which tonal system is used and you will easily identify the product you require.

To replace the red and orange (fill) for a large area of hair use this formula and technique:

Depending on the length and thickness of the hair, take between 1-15ml of the mix tone (average thickness shoulder length hair will require about 8ml) and mix with 60ml of warm water.

Wearing gloves apply the mixture to dry hair, with a brush to the artificially coloured part (not virgin hair) and allow the product to absorb into the hair for 10 minutes.

Blot to remove any excess with an old towel or cotton wool.

Dry on a cool to medium heat.

Apply your target shade (level 6) tint, from root to ends and process as normal.

Do not chose an ash tone for this level of colour, it will neutralise the red in your mix tone and your colour will come out looking uneven and muddy. It's better to use warmer shades of gold and red as they will give a much more natural effect.

If you are adding a brown (dark) tinted light into blonde porous hair, your mix tone should be added into the tint you are using for that particular light. Follow the mixing instructions in your colour chart to make sure you use the correct amount.

Brunettes Check-list

Is the client going brunette from dark or blonde?

If previously coloured blonde, check which colours are missing from the hair and need to be added back.

If going brown from darker, make sure that it is virgin hair as a general rule, tint does not lift tint.

REDS

As with most of the other colours we have looked at, the best candidate for red is in the mid-range around levels 5 - 7. Below level 5 red is a bit more mahogany in tone and above 7 the hair receives more of a copper tone. A good way to see which levels are best suited to a particular colour type i.e. blondes, reds or brunettes, is, take your colour chart and see where the most tonal swatches are concentrated. The manufacturers want to make more of the popular colours within their range. That means that the most popular colours are the best suited because that is what makes them popular. It doesn't mean that hair outside of levels 5 - 7 can't have red; it just means that results won't be quite as good.

Once again it is important to determine if there is any previous colour on the hair and what it is. If there is previous dark tint, we know that in general, we can't lift the hair with tint so we will need to use bleach to lift the colour out and then tone the hair. It may be preferable to use bleach highlights to break up the existing colour and then use a toner of our target shade of red to finish the colour. If you are dealing with naturally dark hair then you will need to check your colour chart to see how many levels of lift you can achieve with the different percentages of hydrogen peroxide. Remember that using normal tint you will only get a maximum lift of 3 levels using 12% hydrogen peroxide. That means if you are working with a natural level 3 virgin hair, you will only achieve a level 6 red (or any other colour for that matter). As it happens most of the popular reds are at level 6, as when you get above this level they start to become more coppery looking, which is often interpreted by the client as ginger. To achieve a colour above level 6 from a natural level 3, you will need to pre-lighten the hair. This is done with bleach but instead of attempting to get to a pale yellow (blonde) pick a level where the exposed contributing pigment is close to what you would see at the level you are targeting. Then when you apply your target colour you

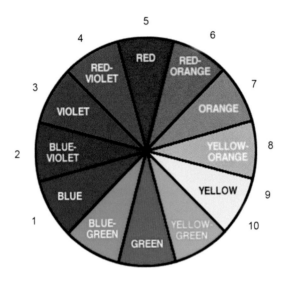

Colour wheel showing residual colours after lifting to a specific level

will be able to choose a tone that enhances rather than neutralises. So, in this case you would take your colour wheel and instead of looking for the opposite colour you would look towards the colours to the sides of your target level.

You could add enhancing tone from yellow/orange to violet. The closer you stay to your target level the stronger the colour will be.

It is quite rare for a natural blonde to change their colour to something either dark or red, therefore, almost all customers wanting to go red from blonde will have artificially coloured hair. So, when we are dealing with colour levels in the upper region i.e. pale blondes levels 8 - 10 or white hair be aware that these colours do not have a much base in them, in fact with white hair there is no base at all. In other words, there is little or no contributing pigment coming from the hair. It will lose its natural look because the hair is not contributing to the colour. This is why we say that the best candidates are within the mid-range of levels because this is where the contributing reds and oranges are. It should also be said that artificially lightened hair is likely to be more porous and therefore the colour will either fade quickly or be expelled by the hair at the first wash, making the quality of your work look inferior.

The way to a successful red is make sure that you have the right customer - one with hair at a level that will give sufficient contributing pigment. Avoid putting strong reds on those with pale yellow or white hair as you will only see the artificial colour that you are applying. Next ensure that you chose the right tint for the job - use your colour wheel and shade chart to find a colour that will enhance the underlying colour at the customer's natural level, helping you to achieve your target colour.

Reds Checklist:

Best candidates for red are levels 3-7.

Check for porosity and any previous colour.

To achieve a successful red, make sure you have the right customer.

POROSITY

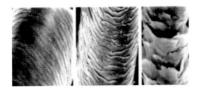

A resistant hair, a normal hair and a porous hair

Porosity is the hair's ability to absorb and retain moisture. The level of porosity in the hair will have a direct bearing on the absorption and longevity of the colour we apply. Think of the hair as if it were a sponge. A smooth man-made sponge with very small holes would represent resistant hair, whilst a

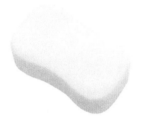 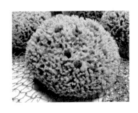

natural sea sponge with lots of large holes would represent porous hair. A normal hair will be somewhere in-between. The more damaged the hair is, the more porous and drier it will be. This is because the damage creates large holes in the hair, which allow the moisture and in our case colour granules to fall out of the hair, causing fade.

Depending how severe the porosity is, we can correct the problem by either adding the missing tone by adding special mix/mix-tone into our formula or we would use the special mix/mix-tone filler as described on page 61.

Resistant hair is very smooth and shiny, so the moisture and colour granules don't fall out easily. However, it is also more difficult to get colour into resistant hair, as the cuticle is completely flat. Use heat and extra time to aid processing.

Porosity Checklist:

Always check for porosity at the consultation.

Think of hair like a sponge, small holes will hold moisture and colour; large holes will allow moisture and colour to escape.

DEVELOPERS AND MIXING

Mixing colour is often thought to be unimportant and a task that should be passed over to an apprentice to complete. In reality, mixing colour is every bit as important as creating the formula and the application technique. All three elements are required and all have to be performed equally well for the colour to succeed. Never pre-prepare your formula as it has a limited life span and should be used as soon as it is mixed. Failure to do this will result in a sub-standard result. The exact measurement of hair colouring products is specific to each manufacturer, you should refer to your manufacturer's instructions for the precise mixing ratio. There are however a number of general aspects that are common to all brands.

Level 1. Semi-permanent colour does not require a developer and can be applied immediately.

Level 2. Quasi or demi permanent colour contains a blend of direct pigments and para-dyes and require low volume hydrogen peroxide for activation. As they are oxidative and contain dye pre-cursors (see Glossary for para-dye) a skin test will be required.

Level 3. Permanent colour is oxidative and requires hydrogen peroxide for activation. These chemicals should only be prepared in a non-metallic bowl as metal reacts badly with hydrogen peroxide. A skin compatibility test is required.

To mix, you will require an electronic weighing scale as hair colour cannot be measured by eye, no matter how much experience the hairdresser has. If an exact colour is required, then exact measurement of the materials is essential. First, place the bowl onto the scale and zero the readout. Next, add your colour pigments to the bowl and weigh out the precise amount you require, finally add your hydrogen peroxide. Here you will need to refer to your manufacturer's instructions to get the exact ratio, it's usually 1:1 but some are 1:1.5 and high lift blondes are usually 1:2. Now mix with a plastic applicator brush until a smooth paste is achieved (no lumps or your colour will be uneven) and allow to stand briefly in order for the solution to stabilise. Bleaches are mixed in a similar way, though may be cream or powder based, again refer to your manufacturer's instructions for the correct ratio of product to developer.

These days most developers are cream based, as they are usually easier to control. Some stylists still prefer to use liquid-based developer but are a minority.

Developers for quasi or demi colours are used at up to 4% usually with a ratio of 1 part colour to 2 parts hydrogen peroxide (check your colour chart). They are not designed to lift and are primarily for depositing colour.

Developers for Level 3 permanent colours are stronger and do lift the colour. Depending on manufacturer, for 1 shade of lift, to stay the same shade or go darker 6% (20 volume) hydrogen peroxide should be used. For 2 shades of lift, use 9% (30 volume) and for 3 shades of lift use 12% (40 volume) hydrogen peroxide. Again, check your manufacturer's instructions for the correct mixing ratio.

Developers and Mixing Check-list:

Always check your manufacturer's recommendations for product to developer ratio.

Make sure you know how much lift each different strength of hydrogen peroxide will give.

Always mix your product into a smooth even paste without lumps.

Use plastic bowls, brushes and clips.

OXIDATION

Here is a little about the science behind a key term often used when discussing hair colourants.

Oxidation is what happens when the oxidising agent hydrogen peroxide is combined with a para-dye (tint cream), creating a new compound.

During the application, the ammonia (alkali) within the mix helps to soften the hair, opening up the cuticle layer and allowing the hydrogen peroxide and dye to enter the cortex, once inside, the hydrogen peroxide chemically changes, increasing the amount of oxygen it contains, giving it a mild bleaching ability which we refer to as lift. **The level of lift is dependent on the strength of the hydrogen peroxide.**

The dye granules then replace the original colour granules that have been removed by the hydrogen peroxide and the new colour is formed.

Oxidizing bleach works by breaking the **chemical bonds** that make up the **Chromophore (the part of the molecule responsible for its colour).**

Hydrogen peroxide H_2O_2 is often described as water with an extra oxygen atom. This description gives an incorrect impression that the two compounds are similar. However, pure hydrogen peroxide will explode if heated to boiling point, it will cause serious contact burns to the skin and can set other materials alight on contact. As hairdressers we only use it in a dilute form, no stronger than 40 volumes or 12%.

Oxidation Check-list:

Oxidation occurs in hair when the hydrogen peroxide increases the amount of oxygen present. This causes a slight lifting in the hair's natural pigment.

The level of lift depends on the strength of hydrogen peroxide used.

The new colour granules are deposited at the same time as the colour is lifted.

Hairdressers only use dilute hydrogen peroxide.

NOTES AND HISTORIES

In today's modern salons, the use of computer technology is becoming commonplace. With purpose made salon software, we can easily keep notes, ranging from the things said at our consultation through to whether the customer takes sugar in their coffee.

The initial notes we make, should cover the customer's wishes, what we have advised and the general condition of the hair. Make note of any poor-quality work done by a previous salon they have visited.

The history covers the work that we carry out for the customer. What the colours we chose are and why.

Here is a real example of a client history. I used Wella products:

Natural level 7, wants to be 10 with silver tone. Colour is patchy and hair is very porous.

Half head highlights 1x tint to 2x bleach Horizontal placement starting with tint underneath and finishing with bleach on parting. Wants to be more silvery looking so using a toner of 10/16 with 0/81 for tone. Lights taken out as ready. Used 63 foils as I had to make very fine weaves to fill gaps.

Bleach with 3% x 2

Colour touch 10g 7/3 with 1cm 0/34 x 1. Used CT as hair is so porous

Toned with 15g of 10/16 with 1/2cm of 0/81 and 30g Pastel developer, under heat for 5 minutes then combed through again at backwash for 5 more. Result - Excellent.

As you can see, all of the information required for the customer's next appointment has been properly recorded. Without proper history notes you will struggle to re-create your work. You will limit what you can achieve to what you can remember and you will limit your prospects as a professional hair colourist.

Notes and Histories Checklist:

Make note of the things said at your consultation.

Note if there was any poor work from another salon.

Make sure that you keep a full and proper record of all of the work you carried out including the result.

QUICK REFERENCE GUIDE

This part of the book is designed to give you a quick and easy way of accessing the information required to formulate the correct colour for your customer.

The Consultation *Page 5*

Determine if a Skin Test is required

Examine the hair for any pre-existing colour work. If it is poor quality tell the customer.

Check porosity and condition (will the colour hold?)

Determine the percentage of white hair.

Establish the customer's natural colour level and tone. Level is the depth of colour (dark v light) and tone is the amount of warmth or coolness that a colour displays.

Establish how much "Exposed Contributing Pigment" (residual colour) there will be at the level you are looking to create.

Check the skin tone and eye colour, is it warm or cool?

Discuss the customer's requirements and ensure that they know what the result is going to be.

Decide your application technique.

Levels and Tones *Page 10*

"Contributing pigment + Artificial colour = Final result"

Base Colour

The dominant colour in any formulation that gives a shade its overall characteristic.

Level

The degree of lightness or darkness (natural or artificial) in the hair regardless of tone.

Tone

The warmth or coolness of a colour – warm tones reflect light and make the hair appear lighter, cool tones absorb light and appear darker.

Determine the natural base colour and tone (Starting Point) and the desired level and tone (End Result)

There are 10 natural levels of hair colour - 1 is Black, 2-5 are Brown (level 2 is darkest brown) 6-10 are Blonde (level 10 is lightest blonde) plus level 12 (high lift).

Contributing pigment, is sometimes called underlying warmth. This underlying warmth is exposed during the lightening process.

Exposed Contributing Pigment, is the colour that is left after the hair has been lifted to a particular level.

The colour can be enhanced or neutralised by choosing the correct tone depending on your desired result.

The Colour Wheel *Page 14*

Understand and use the Colour Wheel.

All colours are made up of Red, Yellow and Blue (Primary Colours).

Opposites on the colour wheel neutralise and give Brown. Neighbouring colours can be used to enhance the tone.

As hair is lifted each level will leave behind a shade of red/yellow called "Exposed Contributing Pigment".

The Numbering System *Page 18*

The slash or dot in-between the numbers on the tube of tint or the shade chart is called a separator.

The numbers to the left of the separator represent the depth of the colour (level). The numbers to the right of the separator describe the tone.

If there is one number to the left of the separator then there is one portion of base.

If the number is doubled e.g. --/ or -- there is a double portion of base.

If there is --/0 or N then these doubles are used to for extra coverage on resistant white hair.

One number to the right of the separator denotes the tone e.g. 6/3 in Wella is level 6 Gold.

Where there are 2 numbers to the right, this shows a dominant and secondary tone, the first is the dominant tone.

Racial Differences in Hair *Page 22*

African hair is thin and almost flat in cross section.

The combination of texture and density of colour granules makes African hair very resistant to artificial colour.

Asian hair is circular in cross section. It is nearly always black and is difficult to lift.

European hair is oval in cross section and has the most varied range of natural textures and colours.

The darker the hair the more difficult it will be to lift without damage.

For the best result, avoid lifting the hair more than 3-4 levels.

Know your end result before you start.

Controlling Warmth *Page 25*

Whenever we lighten hair, we leave behind a residual tone called "Exposed Contributing Pigment".

When we lighten it with tint or bleach, we reveal this residual tone.

Blue has the largest colour molecule and is the easiest to remove and when the blue is gone that only leaves red and yellow, so we see orange.

Red is next, leaving just yellow behind.

Adding Tone *Page 28*

Mix tones are pure tone, use to intensify a colour or correct a tone.

Can be used on pre-bleached hair to create a vivid colour.

Added to toners, can be used to correct unwanted tone e.g. warmth or ash.

Grey Coverage *Page 30*

There is no such thing as an actual grey hair. Non-pigmented hairs are white.

As we age some hair follicles stop producing the pigment melanin which is required to give the hair its colour. Either the individual hairs lose their ability to create pigment and turn white from the base of the hair or they are simply new hairs that do not contain pigment.

Nowadays hair colourant manufacturers refer to their products by levels.

Level 1:

Semi-permanent colour

Level 2:

Quasi semi-permanent sometimes called demi colour

Level 3:

Permanent colourants. These are the most versatile of all hair colourants, they can lighten, stay at the same level or darken the hair and 100% white coverage can be achieved.

2 types of white hair - resistant and non-resistant. Non-resistant white hair is slightly coarse in texture and a little wiry looking; it accepts the colour quite readily. Resistant white hair on the other hand is smooth and glossy in appearance and prone to reject the colour.

It's more difficult to get colour into resistant hair.

When covering white hair, it is best to use the natural/neutral family of tints from your colour palette.

Ash when applied to white hair will give off a violet cast, giving the hair a violet tinge.

Determine the amount of white hair present. Up to 25%, 25-50%, 50-75% and 75-100%.

Decide which materials are most appropriate. Level 1 colour (semi-permanent) will not cover much at all, level 2 colour (quasi or demi colour) will cover about 40% and level 3 (permanent) will cover up to 100%.

What previous procedures have been carried out, if any?

How well have any previous services worked?

Do they want to be lighter than their natural colour or darker?

If there is already artificial colour, is it darker or lighter than the natural colour?

What level is it and is it even?

Is there a re-growth?

What is the natural level of the re-growth?

Do you need to use more than one formula to achieve the result you want because of the difference between the artificial colour and the re-growth?

Here are the simple steps that will help you to achieve the best coverage for white/grey hair.

Examine and determine the current state of the customer's hair.

Decide the Desired Level.

Determine the required tone.

You will only achieve 100% coverage of white hair with tint at level 8 and below.

Apply enough product to fully and evenly saturate the hair.

If the hair is particularly resistant, processing with heat is advised to open the cuticle and allow the product to settle into the cortex. Develop for 25 minutes and then allow to cool for 15 minutes before removing.

Blondes *Page 38*

The best candidates for all over blonde are level 7 and above.

It is possible to achieve up to 7 levels of lift with bleach. However, any customer asking for this level of lift should be advised of the potential for damage.

When using bleach, it is always advisable to use the lowest strength peroxide possible.

Bleach is best used on hair at level 5 and darker as from level 6 tint will give a better result with much less damage.

Oxidative tint is where a chosen colour and tone are applied to the hair which is lifted to the desired level and either neutralising or enhancing tone is created at the same time.

The strength of hydrogen peroxide will determine the level of lift that can be achieved.

High lift blonde colours can lift up to 5 levels to get darker hair up to level 10.

Don't attempt to take a customer from level 2 or 3 up to level 9 or 10, the residual warmth will be too dominant.

Brunettes *Page 40*

The second most common human hair colour.

Whenever we use neutralising colours in our formulations to control warmth, we are creating brown.

The Stages of Lift. Beginning with our starting level the hair goes through red, red/orange, orange, yellow/orange (gold), yellow and pale yellow.

To take the hair back from yellow to brown we must replace the missing colours.

Reds *Page 44*

The best candidate for red is in the mid-range of the colour levels, around levels 3 – 7.

If there is previous dark tint, we know that we can't lift the hair using tint, so, we will need to use bleach to lift the colour out and then tone the hair.

Using normal tint on virgin hair you will only get a maximum lift of three levels using 12% Hydrogen Peroxide.

Almost all customers wanting to go red from blonde will have artificially coloured hair.

Pale blondes and white hair give almost no contributing pigment.

Artificially lightened hair is likely to be more porous.

Porosity *Page 47*

Porosity is the hair's ability to absorb and retain moisture.

Think of the hair as if it were a sponge.

The more damaged the hair is, the more porous and drier it will be.

Colour granules fall out of porous hair more easily causing fade.

Developers and Mixing *Page 49*

Mixing colour is just as important as creating the formula and the application technique.

Never pre-mix your formula.

Refer to the manufacturer's instructions for the precise mixing ratio.

Use a weighing scale as hair colour cannot be measured by eye.

Developers for quasi or semi-permanent colours are used at up to 4%.

Developers for level 3 permanent tint are stronger and do lift the colour.

Oxidation *Page 52*

Oxidation happens when Hydrogen Peroxide is combined with tint cream, creating a new compound which both removes and deposits colour at the same time.

The Ammonia (alkali) within the mix, helps to soften the hair and open the cuticle layer.

Hydrogen Peroxide enters the hair shaft and removes the natural colour through a mild bleaching action, caused by an increase in Oxygen.

Notes and Histories *Page 54*

Notes should cover the customer's wishes, our advice and the general condition of the hair.

Make note of any poor-quality work carried out by a previous salon they have visited.

The history should cover all work you carry out for the customer in detail.

Make sure that your notes are accurate and cover all of the information required.

GLOSSARY

ACID

A liquid which is usually corrosive, with a pH lower than 7. The opposite of an Alkali.

ACTIVATOR

Otherwise called developer, a chemical usually hydrogen peroxide, that is mixed with tint or bleach to oxidise colour from hair.

ACTIVE INGREDIENT

The substance which, contained in a product, actually does the main part of the work that the product is used for.

ALKALI

A liquid with a pH higher than 7. Used in hair tint to soften and open the cuticle, preparing the hair for oxidisation.

ALLERGY

A bodily reaction to an irritant. Skin allergies can be made worse by solutions put on the skin or scalp.

BASIC SHADE

A natural or neutral colour.

BLEACH

A product used to lighten hair by oxidisation, when mixed with hydrogen peroxide.

BLONDE

Hair with a pale, yellow appearance. It contains more Phaeomelanin and is naturally more common in children than adults.

BRASSY

Unflattering warm tones in hair colour caused by chemicals or damage.

CONTRIBUTING PIGMENT

This is the colour that is left behind after the hair has been lightened to a specific level.

CORTEX

The cortex is the main structure of the hair shaft. The cortex determines the colour and texture of the hair.

CUTICLE

The hair cuticles form a protective layer which covers the shaft of hair. They are naturally flat and overlap like scales. To colour hair, they must be opened in order to allow access to the cortex.

DEPTH

The darkness or lightness of a colour.

DEVELOPER

Hydrogen Peroxide

DESIRED COLOUR

Otherwise known as target colour. This is the level and tone that you are aiming to achieve.

GREY HAIR

Correctly known as white hair or non-pigmented hair.

HYDROGEN PEROXIDE

Used to oxidise (lighten) natural colour pigment and to allow for the deposit of artificial colour molecules.

MEDULLA

The medulla is a central zone of cells usually only present in large thick hairs.

NEUTRALISE

To cancel or reduce effect. In the case of hair colouring opposites on the colour wheel will neutralise each other creating brown.

OXIDATION COLOUR

A colour which requires oxygen to make it work. In hair colour oxidation is made possible by hydrogen peroxide.

PARA DYE

Is short for Paraphenylenediamine. It is the ingredient that can cause allergic reactions to hair colour.

PATCH TEST

A test performed in our case with a hair dye on the skin at least 48 hours before its use to determine sensitivity. Also called a skin compatibility test.

PERMANENT COLOUR

Colour which does not wash out.

PIGMENT

Colour.

POROSITY

The ability to absorb and retain moisture.

RESISTANT HAIR

Hair that has a completely closed cuticle making it difficult to accept colour.

SEMI-PERMANENT

A colour which lasts from 4 - 6 shampoos.

TARGET COLOUR

The same as desired colour

TEMPORARY COLOUR

A hair colour that lasts only until you next shampoo your hair.

TINT

Artificial hair colour, can be quasi or semi-permanent or permanent. Requires hydrogen peroxide.

TERTIARY

Third in order. In the case of hair colour, it is the result of mixing a primary (first) colour with a secondary (second) colour, creating a new colour which is a mixture of the other two.

Made in the USA
Middletown, DE
30 March 2023